I0554663

This planner belongs to :

_____

© Copyright by Happy Oak Tree Press. All rights reserved.

Twenty-four

January

S	M	T	W	T	F	S
	1	2	3	4	5	6
7	8	9	10	11	12	13
14	15	16	17	18	19	20
21	22	23	24	25	26	27
28	29	30	31			

February

S	M	T	W	T	F	S
				1	2	3
4	5	6	7	8	9	10
11	12	13	14	15	16	17
18	19	20	21	22	23	24
25	26	27	28	29		

March

S	M	T	W	T	F	S
					1	2
3	4	5	6	7	8	9
10	11	12	13	14	15	16
17	18	19	20	21	22	23
24	25	26	27	28	29	30
31						

April

S	M	T	W	T	F	S
	1	2	3	4	5	6
7	8	9	10	11	12	13
14	15	16	17	18	19	20
21	22	23	24	25	26	27
28	29	30				

May

S	M	T	W	T	F	S
			1	2	3	4
5	6	7	8	9	10	11
12	13	14	15	16	17	18
19	20	21	22	23	24	25
26	27	28	29	30	31	

June

S	M	T	W	T	F	S
						1
2	3	4	5	6	7	8
9	10	11	12	13	14	15
16	17	18	19	20	21	22
23	24	25	26	27	28	29
30						

July

S	M	T	W	T	F	S
	1	2	3	4	5	6
7	8	9	10	11	12	13
14	15	16	17	18	19	20
21	22	23	24	25	26	27
28	29	30	31			

August

S	M	T	W	T	F	S
				1	2	3
4	5	6	7	8	9	10
11	12	13	14	15	16	17
18	19	20	21	22	23	24
25	26	27	28	29	30	31

September

S	M	T	W	T	F	S
1	2	3	4	5	6	7
8	9	10	11	12	13	14
15	16	17	18	19	20	21
22	23	24	25	26	27	28
29	30					

October

S	M	T	W	T	F	S
		1	2	3	4	5
6	7	8	9	10	11	12
13	14	15	16	17	18	19
20	21	22	23	24	25	26
27	28	29	30	31		

November

S	M	T	W	T	F	S
					1	2
3	4	5	6	7	8	9
10	11	12	13	14	15	16
17	18	19	20	21	22	23
24	25	26	27	28	29	30

December

S	M	T	W	T	F	S
1	2	3	4	5	6	7
8	9	10	11	12	13	14
15	16	17	18	19	20	21
22	23	24	25	26	27	28
29	30	31				

Year in Pixels

	J	F	M	A	M	J	J	A	S	O	N	D
1.												
2.												
3.												
4.												
5.												
6.												
7.												
8.												
9.												
10.												
11.												
12.												
13.												
14.												
15.												
16.												
17.												
18.												
19.												
20.												
21.												
22.												
23.												
24.												
25.												
26.												
27.												
28.												
29.												
30.												
31.												

Color Codes

Notes

January

MONDAY	TUESDAY	WEDNESDAY	THURSDAY
1	2	3	4
8	9	10	11
15	16	17	18
22	23	24	25
29	30	31	

January

FRIDAY	SATURDAY	SUNDAY	NOTES
5	6	7	○
			○
			○
			○
			○
12	13	14	○
			○
			○
			○
19	20	21	○
			○
			○
			○
			○
26	27	28	○
			○
			○
			○
			○
			NOTES

February

MONDAY	TUESDAY	WEDNESDAY	THURSDAY
			1
5	6	7	8
12	13	14	15
19	20	21	22
26	27	28	29

February

FRIDAY	SATURDAY	SUNDAY	NOTES
2	3	4	○
			○
			○
			○
			○
9	10	11	○
			○
			○
			○
			○
16	17	18	○
			○
			○
			○
			○
23	24	25	○
			○
			○
			○
			○
			NOTES

March

MONDAY	TUESDAY	WEDNESDAY	THURSDAY
4	5	6	7
11	12	13	14
18	19	20	21
25	26	27	28

March

FRIDAY	SATURDAY	SUNDAY	NOTES
1	2	3	○
			○
			○
			○
			○
8	9	10	○
			○
			○
			○
			○
15	16	17	○
			○
			○
			○
			○
22	23	24	○
			○
			○
			○
			○
29	30	31	NOTES

April

MONDAY	TUESDAY	WEDNESDAY	THURSDAY
1	2	3	4
8	9	10	11
15	16	17	18
22	23	24	25
29	30		

April

2024

FRIDAY	SATURDAY	SUNDAY	NOTES
5	6	7	○
			○
			○
			○
			○
12	13	14	○
			○
			○
			○
			○
19	20	21	○
			○
			○
			○
			○
26	27	28	○
			○
			○
			○
			○
			NOTES

May

MONDAY	TUESDAY	WEDNESDAY	THURSDAY
		1	2
6	7	8	9
13	14	15	16
20	21	22	23
27	28	29	30

May

FRIDAY	SATURDAY	SUNDAY	NOTES
3	4	5	○
			○
			○
			○
			○
10	11	12	○
			○
			○
			○
			○
17	18	19	○
			○
			○
			○
			○
24	25	26	○
			○
			○
			○
			○
31			NOTES

June

MONDAY	TUESDAY	WEDNESDAY	THURSDAY
3	4	5	6
10	11	12	13
17	18	19	20
24	25	26	27

June

FRIDAY	SATURDAY	SUNDAY	NOTES
	1	2	○
			○
			○
			○
			○
7	8	9	○
			○
			○
			○
			○
14	15	16	○
			○
			○
			○
			○
21	22	23	○
			○
			○
			○
			○
28	29	30	NOTES

July

2024

MONDAY	TUESDAY	WEDNESDAY	THURSDAY
1	2	3	4
8	9	10	11
15	16	17	18
22	23	24	25
29	30	31	

July

FRIDAY	SATURDAY	SUNDAY	NOTES
5	6	7	○
			○
			○
			○
			○
12	13	14	○
			○
			○
			○
			○
19	20	21	○
			○
			○
			○
26	27	28	○
			○
			○
			○
			○
			NOTES

August

MONDAY	TUESDAY	WEDNESDAY	THURSDAY
			1
5	6	7	8
12	13	14	15
19	20	21	22
26	27	28	29

August

FRIDAY	SATURDAY	SUNDAY	NOTES
2	3	4	○
			○
			○
			○
			○
9	10	11	○
			○
			○
			○
16	17	18	○
			○
			○
			○
			○
23	24	25	○
			○
			○
			○
			○
30	31		NOTES

September

MONDAY	TUESDAY	WEDNESDAY	THURSDAY
2	3	4	5
9	10	11	12
16	17	18	19
23	24	25	26

September

FRIDAY	SATURDAY	SUNDAY	NOTES
		1	○
			○
			○
			○
			○
6	7	8	○
			○
			○
			○
13	14	15	○
			○
			○
			○
			○
20	21	22	○
			○
			○
			○
			○
27	28	29	30

October

2024

MONDAY	TUESDAY	WEDNESDAY	THURSDAY
	1	2	3
7	8	9	10
14	15	16	17
21	22	23	24
28	29	30	31

October 2024

FRIDAY	SATURDAY	SUNDAY	NOTES
4	5	6	○
			○
			○
			○
			○
11	12	13	○
			○
			○
			○
			○
18	19	20	○
			○
			○
			○
25	26	27	○
			○
			○
			○
			○
			NOTES

November

MONDAY	TUESDAY	WEDNESDAY	THURSDAY
4	5	6	7
11	12	13	14
18	19	20	21
25	26	27	28

November

2024

FRIDAY	SATURDAY	SUNDAY	NOTES
1	2	3	○
			○
			○
			○
			○
8	9	10	○
			○
			○
			○
15	16	17	○
			○
			○
			○
			○
22	23	24	○
			○
			○
			○
			○
29	30		NOTES

December

MONDAY	TUESDAY	WEDNESDAY	THURSDAY
2	3	4	5
9	10	11	12
16	17	18	19
23	24	25	26

December

FRIDAY	SATURDAY	SUNDAY	NOTES
		1	○
			○
			○
			○
			○
6	7	8	○
			○
			○
			○
13	14	15	○
			○
			○
			○
			○
20	21	22	○
			○
			○
			○
			○
27	28	29	30 / 31

December
2023

01 FRIDAY

02 SATURDAY

03 SUNDAY

04 MONDAY

December
2023

05 TUESDAY

06 WEDNESDAY

07 THURSDAY

08 FRIDAY

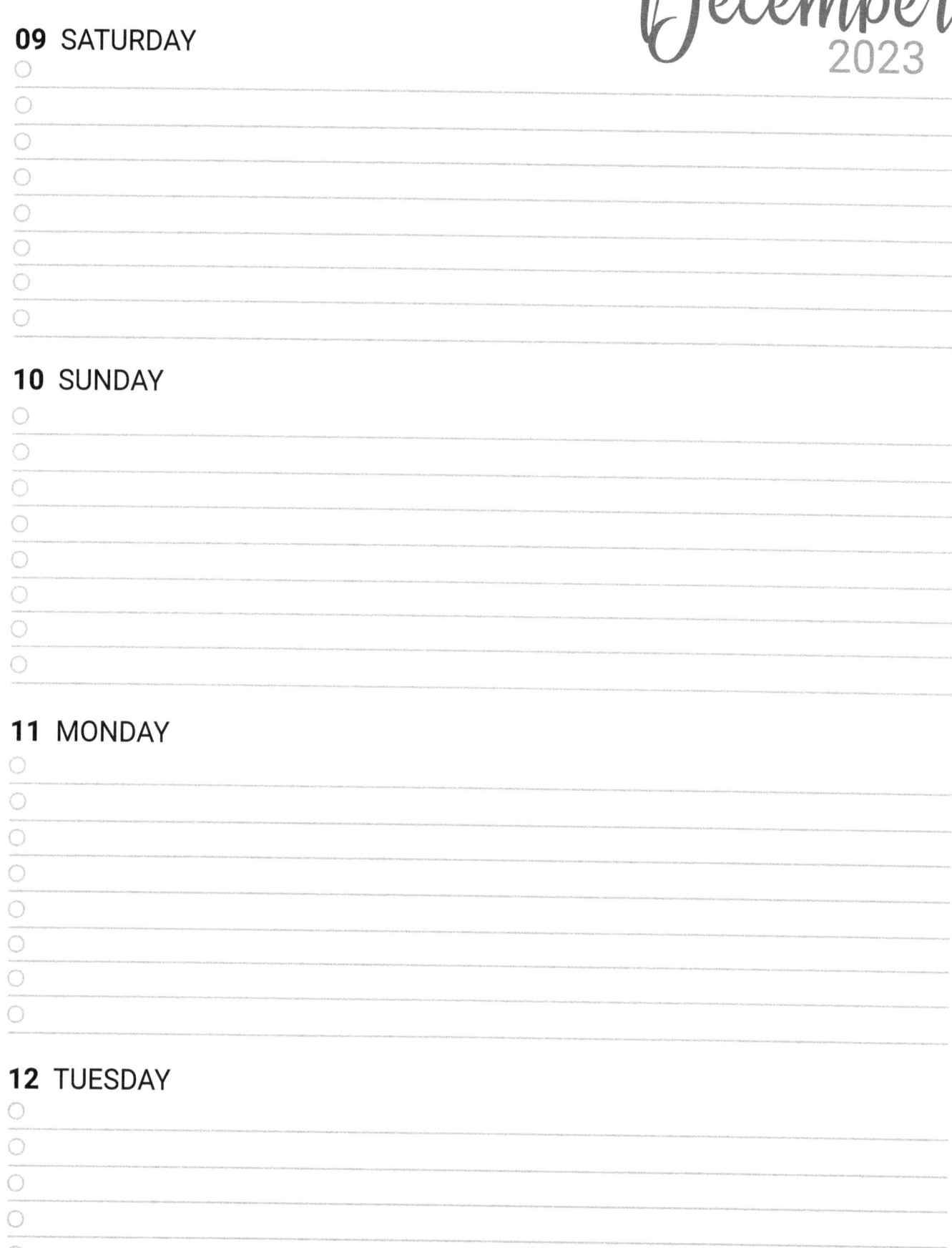

December
2023

09 SATURDAY

10 SUNDAY

11 MONDAY

12 TUESDAY

December
2023

13 WEDNESDAY

14 THURSDAY

15 FRIDAY

16 SATURDAY

December
2023

17 SUNDAY

18 MONDAY

19 TUESDAY

20 WEDNESDAY

21 THURSDAY

22 FRIDAY

23 SATURDAY

24 SUNDAY

December
2023

25 MONDAY

26 TUESDAY

27 WEDNESDAY

28 THURSDAY

December
2023

29 FRIDAY

30 SATURDAY

31 SUNDAY

NOTES

January
2024

01 MONDAY

- ○
- ○
- ○
- ○
- ○
- ○
- ○
- ○

02 TUESDAY

- ○
- ○
- ○
- ○
- ○
- ○
- ○
- ○

03 WEDNESDAY

- ○
- ○
- ○
- ○
- ○
- ○
- ○
- ○

04 THURSDAY

- ○
- ○
- ○
- ○
- ○

05 FRIDAY

○
○
○
○
○
○
○
○

06 SATURDAY

○
○
○
○
○
○
○
○

07 SUNDAY

○
○
○
○
○
○
○
○

08 MONDAY

○
○
○
○
○

09 TUESDAY

○ ....
○ ....
○ ....
○ ....
○ ....
○ ....
○ ....
○ ....

10 WEDNESDAY

○ ....
○ ....
○ ....
○ ....
○ ....
○ ....
○ ....
○ ....

11 THURSDAY

○ ....
○ ....
○ ....
○ ....
○ ....
○ ....
○ ....
○ ....

12 FRIDAY

○ ....
○ ....
○ ....
○ ....
○ ....

13 SATURDAY

14 SUNDAY

15 MONDAY

16 TUESDAY

17 WEDNESDAY

○
○
○
○
○
○
○
○

18 THURSDAY

○
○
○
○
○
○
○
○

19 FRIDAY

○
○
○
○
○
○
○
○

20 SATURDAY

○
○
○
○
○

21 SUNDAY

○
○
○
○
○
○
○
○

22 MONDAY

○
○
○
○
○
○
○
○

23 TUESDAY

○
○
○
○
○
○
○
○

24 WEDNESDAY

○
○
○
○
○

25 THURSDAY

○
○
○
○
○
○
○
○

26 FRIDAY

○
○
○
○
○
○
○
○

27 SATURDAY

○
○
○
○
○
○
○
○

28 SUNDAY

○
○
○
○
○

29 MONDAY

30 TUESDAY

31 WEDNESDAY

NOTES

February
2024

01 THURSDAY

○
○
○
○
○
○
○
○

02 FRIDAY

○
○
○
○
○
○
○
○

03 SATURDAY

○
○
○
○
○
○
○
○

04 SUNDAY

○
○
○
○
○

February
2024

05 MONDAY

06 TUESDAY

07 WEDNESDAY

08 THURSDAY

09 FRIDAY

10 SATURDAY

11 SUNDAY

12 MONDAY

February 2024

13 TUESDAY

14 WEDNESDAY

15 THURSDAY

16 FRIDAY

17 SATURDAY

18 SUNDAY

19 MONDAY

20 TUESDAY

February
2024

21 WEDNESDAY

22 THURSDAY

23 FRIDAY

24 SATURDAY

25 SUNDAY

26 MONDAY

27 TUESDAY

28 WEDNESDAY

29 THURSDAY

○ _____
○ _____
○ _____
○ _____
○ _____
○ _____
○ _____
○ _____

NOTES

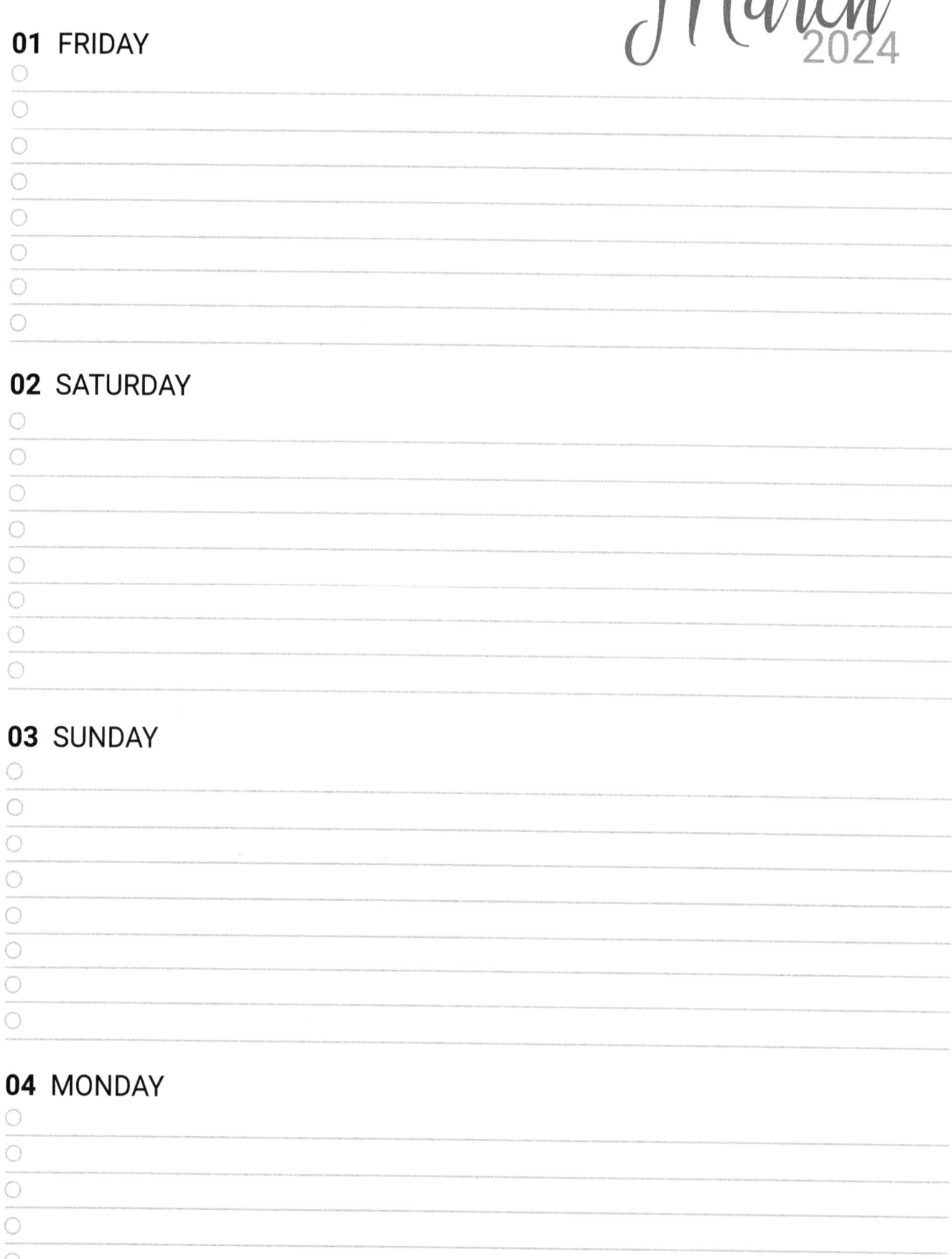

March
2024

01 FRIDAY

02 SATURDAY

03 SUNDAY

04 MONDAY

05 TUESDAY

○
○
○
○
○
○
○
○

06 WEDNESDAY

○
○
○
○
○
○
○
○

07 THURSDAY

○
○
○
○
○
○
○
○

08 FRIDAY

○
○
○
○
○

March 2024

09 SATURDAY

10 SUNDAY

11 MONDAY

12 TUESDAY

13 WEDNESDAY

14 THURSDAY

15 FRIDAY

16 SATURDAY

March 2024

17 SUNDAY

18 MONDAY

19 TUESDAY

20 WEDNESDAY

21 THURSDAY

○ _____
○ _____
○ _____
○ _____
○ _____
○ _____
○ _____
○ _____

22 FRIDAY

○ _____
○ _____
○ _____
○ _____
○ _____
○ _____
○ _____
○ _____

23 SATURDAY

○ _____
○ _____
○ _____
○ _____
○ _____
○ _____
○ _____
○ _____

24 SUNDAY

○ _____
○ _____
○ _____
○ _____
○ _____

25 MONDAY

26 TUESDAY

27 WEDNESDAY

28 THURSDAY

March 2024

29 FRIDAY

○
○
○
○
○
○
○
○

30 SATURDAY

○
○
○
○
○
○
○
○

31 SUNDAY

○
○
○
○
○
○
○
○

NOTES

April
2024

01 MONDAY

02 TUESDAY

03 WEDNESDAY

04 THURSDAY

April
2024

05 FRIDAY

○
○
○
○
○
○
○
○

06 SATURDAY

○
○
○
○
○
○
○
○

07 SUNDAY

○
○
○
○
○
○
○
○

08 MONDAY

○
○
○
○
○

09 TUESDAY

10 WEDNESDAY

11 THURSDAY

12 FRIDAY

13 SATURDAY

14 SUNDAY

15 MONDAY

16 TUESDAY

April
2024

17 WEDNESDAY

18 THURSDAY

19 FRIDAY

20 SATURDAY

April
2024

21 SUNDAY

○
○
○
○
○
○
○
○

22 MONDAY

○
○
○
○
○
○
○
○

23 TUESDAY

○
○
○
○
○
○
○
○

24 WEDNESDAY

○
○
○
○
○

April
2024

25 THURSDAY

26 FRIDAY

27 SATURDAY

28 SUNDAY

April
2024

29 MONDAY

○
○
○
○
○
○
○
○

30 TUESDAY

○
○
○
○
○
○
○
○

NOTES

01 WEDNESDAY

02 THURSDAY

03 FRIDAY

04 SATURDAY

05 SUNDAY

06 MONDAY

07 TUESDAY

08 WEDNESDAY

May 2024

09 THURSDAY

10 FRIDAY

11 SATURDAY

12 SUNDAY

13 MONDAY

14 TUESDAY

15 WEDNESDAY

16 THURSDAY

17 FRIDAY

18 SATURDAY

19 SUNDAY

20 MONDAY

21 TUESDAY
- ○
- ○
- ○
- ○
- ○
- ○
- ○
- ○

22 WEDNESDAY
- ○
- ○
- ○
- ○
- ○
- ○
- ○
- ○

23 THURSDAY
- ○
- ○
- ○
- ○
- ○
- ○
- ○
- ○

24 FRIDAY
- ○
- ○
- ○
- ○
- ○

May
2024

25 SATURDAY

26 SUNDAY

27 MONDAY

28 TUESDAY

29 WEDNESDAY

○
○
○
○
○
○
○
○

30 THURSDAY

○
○
○
○
○
○
○
○

31 FRIDAY

○
○
○
○
○
○
○
○

NOTES

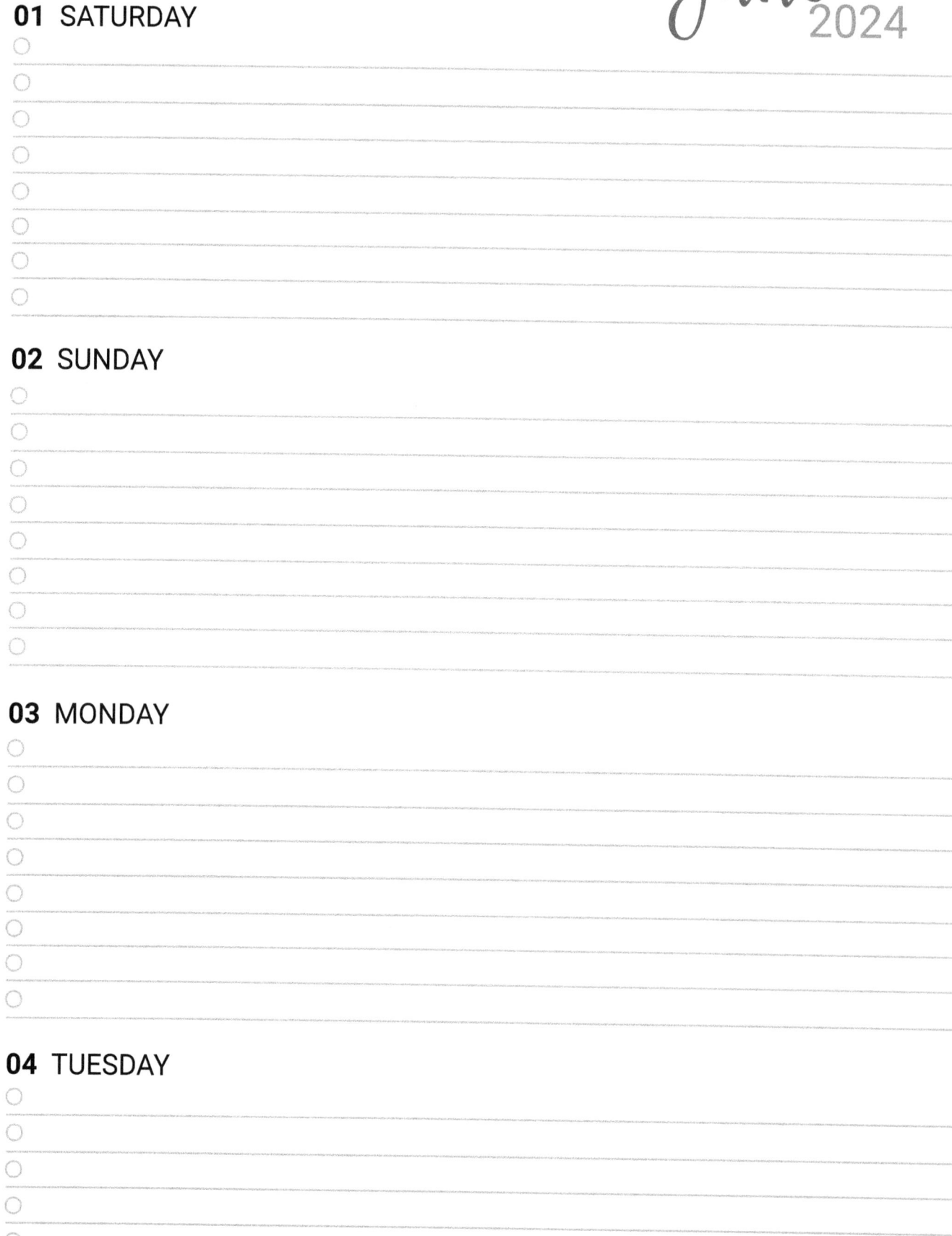

June 2024

01 SATURDAY

02 SUNDAY

03 MONDAY

04 TUESDAY

05 WEDNESDAY

06 THURSDAY

07 FRIDAY

08 SATURDAY

09 SUNDAY

○
○
○
○
○
○
○
○

10 MONDAY

○
○
○
○
○
○
○
○

11 TUESDAY

○
○
○
○
○
○
○
○

12 WEDNESDAY

○
○
○
○

13 THURSDAY

○
○
○
○
○
○
○
○

14 FRIDAY

○
○
○
○
○
○
○
○

15 SATURDAY

○
○
○
○
○
○
○
○

16 SUNDAY

○
○
○
○
○

June 2024

17 MONDAY

18 TUESDAY

19 WEDNESDAY

20 THURSDAY

June 2024

21 FRIDAY

○
○
○
○
○
○
○
○

22 SATURDAY

○
○
○
○
○
○
○
○

23 SUNDAY

○
○
○
○
○
○
○
○

24 MONDAY

○
○
○
○
○

25 TUESDAY

26 WEDNESDAY

27 THURSDAY

28 FRIDAY

29 SATURDAY

○ _____
○ _____
○ _____
○ _____
○ _____
○ _____
○ _____
○ _____

30 SUNDAY

○ _____
○ _____
○ _____
○ _____
○ _____
○ _____
○ _____
○ _____

NOTES

_____
_____
_____
_____
_____
_____
_____
_____
_____
_____
_____

01 MONDAY

○
○
○
○
○
○
○
○

02 TUESDAY

○
○
○
○
○
○
○
○

03 WEDNESDAY

○
○
○
○
○
○
○
○

04 THURSDAY

○
○
○
○
○

05 FRIDAY

○
○
○
○
○
○
○

06 SATURDAY

○
○
○
○
○
○
○
○

07 SUNDAY

○
○
○
○
○
○
○

08 MONDAY

○
○
○
○
○

09 TUESDAY

○
○
○
○
○
○
○
○

10 WEDNESDAY

○
○
○
○
○
○
○
○

11 THURSDAY

○
○
○
○
○
○
○
○

12 FRIDAY

○
○
○
○
○

13 SATURDAY

14 SUNDAY

15 MONDAY

16 TUESDAY

17 WEDNESDAY

18 THURSDAY

19 FRIDAY

20 SATURDAY

21 SUNDAY

22 MONDAY

23 TUESDAY

24 WEDNESDAY

25 THURSDAY

○
○
○
○
○
○
○
○

26 FRIDAY

○
○
○
○
○
○
○
○

27 SATURDAY

○
○
○
○
○
○
○
○

28 SUNDAY

○
○
○
○
○

29 MONDAY

○
○
○
○
○
○
○
○

30 TUESDAY

○
○
○
○
○
○
○
○

31 WEDNESDAY

○
○
○
○
○
○
○
○

NOTES

August
2024

01 THURSDAY

02 FRIDAY

03 SATURDAY

04 SUNDAY

August
2024

05 MONDAY

○ _____
○ _____
○ _____
○ _____
○ _____
○ _____
○ _____
○ _____

06 TUESDAY

○ _____
○ _____
○ _____
○ _____
○ _____
○ _____
○ _____
○ _____

07 WEDNESDAY

○ _____
○ _____
○ _____
○ _____
○ _____
○ _____
○ _____
○ _____

08 THURSDAY

○ _____
○ _____
○ _____
○ _____
○ _____

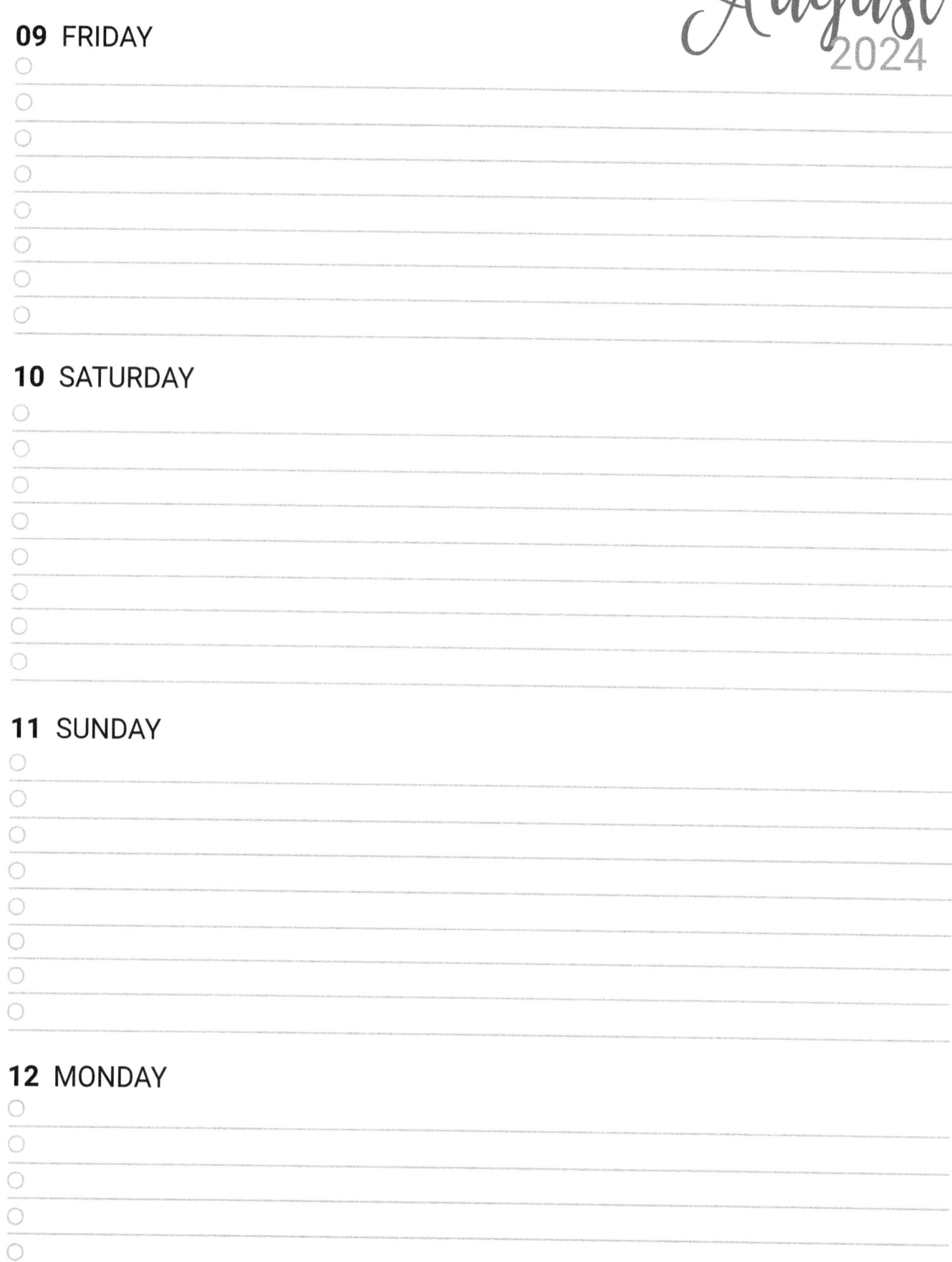

August
2024

09 FRIDAY

10 SATURDAY

11 SUNDAY

12 MONDAY

13 TUESDAY

14 WEDNESDAY

15 THURSDAY

16 FRIDAY

17 SATURDAY
- ○
- ○
- ○
- ○
- ○
- ○
- ○
- ○

18 SUNDAY
- ○
- ○
- ○
- ○
- ○
- ○
- ○
- ○

19 MONDAY
- ○
- ○
- ○
- ○
- ○
- ○
- ○
- ○

20 TUESDAY
- ○
- ○
- ○
- ○
- ○

August 2024

21 WEDNESDAY

○ _____
○ _____
○ _____
○ _____
○ _____
○ _____
○ _____
○ _____

22 THURSDAY

○ _____
○ _____
○ _____
○ _____
○ _____
○ _____
○ _____
○ _____

23 FRIDAY

○ _____
○ _____
○ _____
○ _____
○ _____
○ _____
○ _____
○ _____

24 SATURDAY

○ _____
○ _____
○ _____
○ _____
○ _____

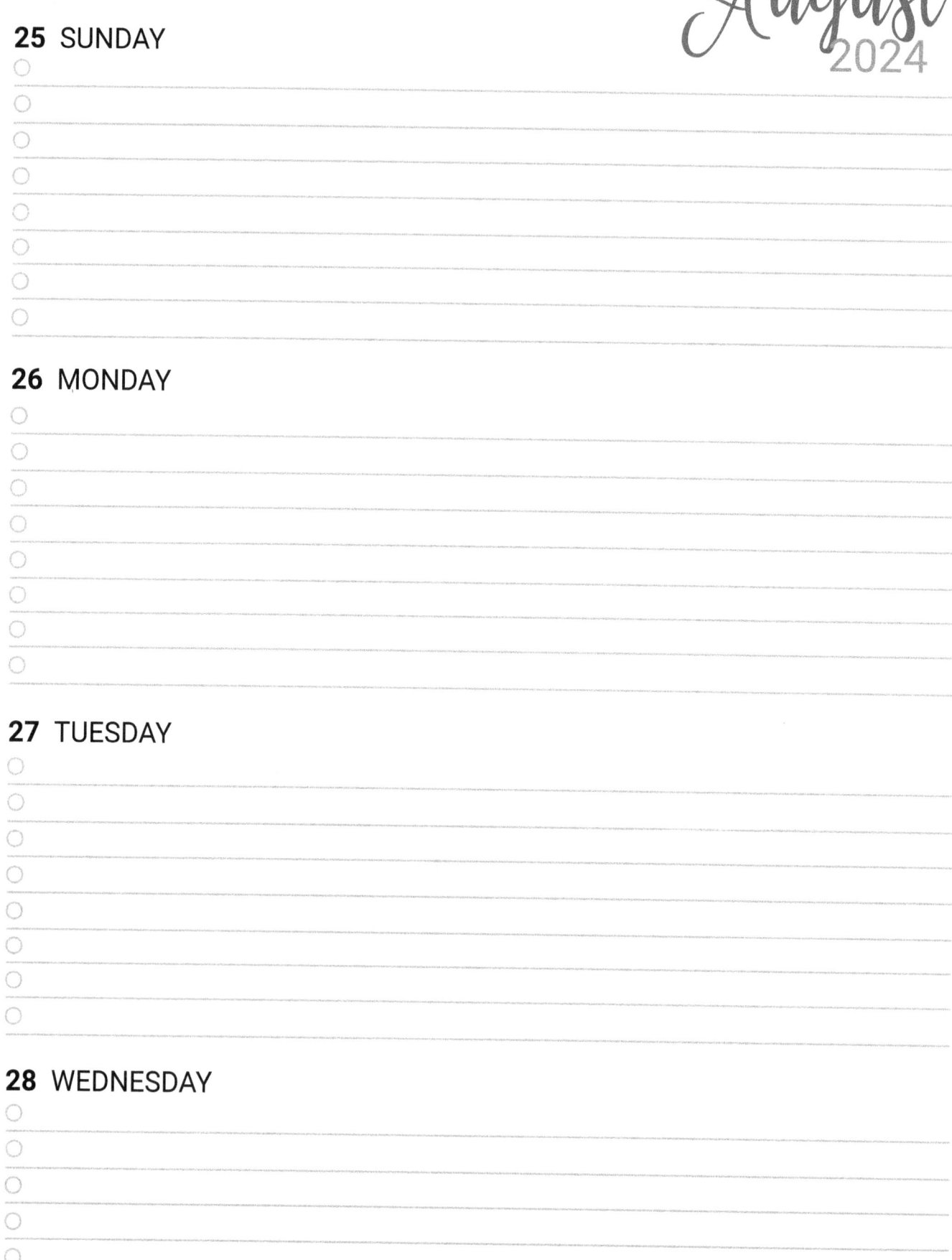

August
2024

25 SUNDAY

26 MONDAY

27 TUESDAY

28 WEDNESDAY

29 THURSDAY

30 FRIDAY

31 SATURDAY

NOTES

01 SUNDAY

○
○
○
○
○
○
○
○

02 MONDAY

○
○
○
○
○
○
○
○

03 TUESDAY

○
○
○
○
○
○
○
○

04 WEDNESDAY

○
○
○
○

05 THURSDAY

○ _____
○ _____
○ _____
○ _____
○ _____
○ _____
○ _____
○ _____

06 FRIDAY

○ _____
○ _____
○ _____
○ _____
○ _____
○ _____
○ _____
○ _____

07 SATURDAY

○ _____
○ _____
○ _____
○ _____
○ _____
○ _____
○ _____
○ _____

08 SUNDAY

○ _____
○ _____
○ _____
○ _____
○ _____

09 MONDAY

○
○
○
○
○
○
○
○

10 TUESDAY

○
○
○
○
○
○
○
○

11 WEDNESDAY

○
○
○
○
○
○
○
○

12 THURSDAY

○
○
○
○
○

13 FRIDAY

14 SATURDAY

15 SUNDAY

16 MONDAY

17 TUESDAY

18 WEDNESDAY

19 THURSDAY

20 FRIDAY

21 SATURDAY

○
○
○
○
○
○
○
○

22 SUNDAY

○
○
○
○
○
○
○
○

23 MONDAY

○
○
○
○
○
○
○
○

24 TUESDAY

○
○
○
○
○

25 WEDNESDAY

26 THURSDAY

27 FRIDAY

28 SATURDAY

29 SUNDAY

- ○
- ○
- ○
- ○
- ○
- ○
- ○
- ○

30 MONDAY

- ○
- ○
- ○
- ○
- ○
- ○
- ○
- ○

NOTES

October
2024

01 TUESDAY

02 WEDNESDAY

03 THURSDAY

04 FRIDAY

October
2024

05 SATURDAY

○ _____
○ _____
○ _____
○ _____
○ _____
○ _____
○ _____
○ _____

06 SUNDAY

○ _____
○ _____
○ _____
○ _____
○ _____
○ _____
○ _____
○ _____

07 MONDAY

○ _____
○ _____
○ _____
○ _____
○ _____
○ _____
○ _____
○ _____

08 TUESDAY

○ _____
○ _____
○ _____
○ _____
○ _____

09 WEDNESDAY

10 THURSDAY

11 FRIDAY

12 SATURDAY

October
2024

13 SUNDAY

14 MONDAY

15 TUESDAY

16 WEDNESDAY

17 THURSDAY

18 FRIDAY

19 SATURDAY

20 SUNDAY

October
2024

21 MONDAY

○
○
○
○
○
○
○
○

22 TUESDAY

○
○
○
○
○
○
○
○

23 WEDNESDAY

○
○
○
○
○
○
○
○

24 THURSDAY

○
○
○
○
○

25 FRIDAY

○

○

○

○

○

○

○

○

26 SATURDAY

○

○

○

○

○

○

○

○

27 SUNDAY

○

○

○

○

○

○

○

○

28 MONDAY

○

○

○

○

○

October
2024

29 TUESDAY

○
○
○
○
○
○
○
○

30 WEDNESDAY

○
○
○
○
○
○
○
○

31 THURSDAY

○
○
○
○
○
○
○
○

NOTES

01 FRIDAY

○
○
○
○
○
○
○
○

02 SATURDAY

○
○
○
○
○
○
○
○

03 SUNDAY

○
○
○
○
○
○
○
○

04 MONDAY

○
○
○
○
○

05 TUESDAY

06 WEDNESDAY

07 THURSDAY

08 FRIDAY

09 SATURDAY

10 SUNDAY

11 MONDAY

12 TUESDAY

13 WEDNESDAY

14 THURSDAY

15 FRIDAY

16 SATURDAY

November
2024

17 SUNDAY

18 MONDAY

19 TUESDAY

20 WEDNESDAY

21 THURSDAY

22 FRIDAY

23 SATURDAY

24 SUNDAY

25 MONDAY

○
○
○
○
○
○
○
○

26 TUESDAY

○
○
○
○
○
○
○
○

27 WEDNESDAY

○
○
○
○
○
○
○
○

28 THURSDAY

○
○
○
○
○

29 FRIDAY

- ○
- ○
- ○
- ○
- ○
- ○
- ○
- ○

30 SATURDAY

- ○
- ○
- ○
- ○
- ○
- ○
- ○
- ○

NOTES

December
2024

01 SUNDAY

02 MONDAY

03 TUESDAY

04 WEDNESDAY

December
2024

05 THURSDAY

○
○
○
○
○
○
○
○

06 FRIDAY

○
○
○
○
○
○
○
○

07 SATURDAY

○
○
○
○
○
○
○
○

08 SUNDAY

○
○
○
○
○

09 MONDAY

10 TUESDAY

11 WEDNESDAY

12 THURSDAY

13 FRIDAY

14 SATURDAY

15 SUNDAY

16 MONDAY

December
2024

17 TUESDAY

18 WEDNESDAY

19 THURSDAY

20 FRIDAY

December
2024

21 SATURDAY

22 SUNDAY

23 MONDAY

24 TUESDAY

25 WEDNESDAY

○
○
○
○
○
○
○
○

26 THURSDAY

○
○
○
○
○
○
○
○

27 FRIDAY

○
○
○
○
○
○
○
○

28 SATURDAY

○
○
○
○
○

December
2024

29 SUNDAY

30 MONDAY

31 TUESDAY

NOTES

www.ingramcontent.com/pod-product-compliance
Lightning Source LLC
Chambersburg PA
CBHW081332120626
46546CB00011B/3317